AUTISM IN AN AFRICAN AMERICAN FAMILY

Deborah A. Lonzer, M.Ed.

Copyright © 2025 by Deborah A Lonzer, M.Ed.

All rights reserved.

Published in the United States by Kindle Direct Publishing

ISBN: 9798275124118

No part of this publication may be reproduced, stored in a retrieval system, or transmitted in any form or by any means electronic, mechanical, photocopying, recording, or otherwise, without the written permission of the author or publisher.

Acknowledgements

I have so many mothers, grandmothers and cousins who inspired and encouraged me to tell my story. Thank you.

Sissy, I deeply appreciate you in helping me to see who I am through your eyes as a mother, a friend and a compassionate human being.

Thank you Marcia for tenderly walking me through the editing of this sensitive story. Thank you for pushing me to tell more of my truth and to be transparent about my journey with my autistic sons.

Contents:

Why This?	1
When Considering a DIAGNOSIS	4
SUPPORT	6
Extended Family Support	
Siblings	
AT HOME	9
BEHAVIOR	12
MAKING SOCIAL CONTACT	16
CHILDCARE	17
SCHOOL	19
SCHOOL SOCIAL LOSSES	23
Peer Bullying	
Teacher Bullying	
Academic Bullying	
COMMUNITY AGENCIES	29
THE HEART OF THE MATTER	34
A Mother's Heart/Hurt	
How a Mother Feels	
DIVINE GUIDANCE	42
THINGS TO CONSIDER	47

WHY THIS?

This story is for African American families and general readers as well. Autism Spectrum Disorder (ASD) poses a greater challenge for the African American family than for the Caucasian American family. Autism in the African American family is multifaceted. Due to the circumstances that African Americans have endured and survived over and over again, we approach autism through a damaged lens in American society.

If you are reading this you may be wondering about the different experiences of African Americans. You may be curious about the rise of autism. Maybe you simply want to take a look into an African American family's disability issues. Or you may be looking for just a little validation on what you have or are experiencing to assure yourself that you aren't crazy.

As we learn more and more about the signs of autism we can now look to new research, and we may recognize some of the people we knew in the past as being different socially. We've seen socially awkward folks before and weren't sure why they were that way. As African Americans, we have typically hidden or covered for our children's awkwardness, hiding them from social gatherings and attending very few to no public appearances. Church can sometimes be a safe place for a loved one, but not without misunderstanding or even ridicule at times.

We often don't want our children to get tested or evaluated for mental issues and learning problems. Some reasons may be because of the lack of resources in our community or not knowing where to get help for our loved one. Fear is also a big factor when it comes to the evaluation of our loved one:

♦ "Even if I have a diagnosis, then what?"

♦ "We're Black, and life is already hard with the odds stacked against my loved one based upon his/her skin color. Then add to that a label of ASD to increase the odds."

♦ "We just have to work with him more."

♦ "Maybe he'll outgrow 'it'."

In the meantime frustration builds with slow to no progress. Many parents are still determined to "beat this" with hard work, discipline and close attention. The family is bombarded with critiques, putdowns, advice, and are told to read this, watch that, see this doctor, that counselor, etc. When you are so overwhelmed addressing your child's extremely demanding needs, you just don't have the time to read, watch TV, chase down doctors or counselors. We are just spent, seeing no light at the end of the tunnel.

WHEN CONSIDERING A DIAGNOSIS

When my oldest son was eight, we began the very slow process of learning what Asperger Syndrome was. Now what? Medication? Counseling? Where and what? Resources are neither clear nor forthcoming. Some families may just resign themselves to just keep doing what they are doing and hope for the best. African American families are often slow to get a diagnosis for many reasons: pride, shame, the unknown, the, "what's next," economic issues, and fear of not knowing how to live with this issue.[1]

Finding different doctors, counselors, neurologists and psychologists has been a long, and in some cases, a poisonous journey for both of my sons. Their diagnosis of Asperger Syndrome comes with other medical issues (comorbidities): attention deficit, hyperactivity, gastroenterological problems, depression, hypersensitivity, anxiety, and more.

Now the hunt for services and doctors began with the

---

[1] Research now shows that *Black children often get diagnosed later than white children*; the average age of diagnosis for Black children is 5.4 years compared to the national average of 4.9 years. Autism in the Black community is—for the first time—higher than in the non-Hispanic white community.

https://www.autismspeaks.org/blog/autism-in-black-community

hope that help was out there for my sons. I searched for more and more information on how to educate and discipline my children and how to educate educators about this disorder. When my sons were finally diagnosed, only one child in a thousand was diagnosed with ASD. Now that ratio is one in thirty-six, and I had two sons with this condition.

ASD children have great difficulty communicating, primarily due to slow mental processing speed. Sensory issues are also a big part of their frustration, self-soothing, self-injury and isolation. Even with this basic information, there are still no two autistic children that are alike. To add to that, life experiences in the African American culture are as varied as our skin tone.

SUPPORT [2]

Community Agencies Support

Resources just weren't clear nor forthcoming. Professionals weren't giving helpful directions. I felt I just hadn't asked the right questions. Once locating services, if I didn't ask the right questions, no services were available for my family. I found the more I challenged the agencies for resources, I would get a *sprinkle* of support. When I wrote letters, there would be a little bit more of a *sprinkle* of services. At one meeting I inquired about my son's sensory diet that the doctor prescribed. In response, I was told, "since you know what your son needs, why don't you do it with him?" The insensitivity to the needs of my disabled children filled me with such anger in my brain and heart that it left me gasping for air. I retorted back, "If I wasn't able or knowledgeable enough to do what you are saying, what would you do then for my son?" They often had no response.

No one offered to see my child within the setting of his entire family either, as if our needs and our livelihood at

---

[2] "African American children with autism experience racial disparities in timing of diagnosis and access to quality interventions. https://pmc.ncbi.nlm.nih.gov/articles/PMC7461218/

home didn't even exist. I think their goal was to get me to accept "no" without question or further investigation. They just wanted me to go away.

Extended Family Support

Our extended family members work with us as well as they can when it comes to caring for our child. However, most families don't understand the complexities and may even feel afraid.

I took my sons to a family member for a couple of hours and was met at the door with, "Did they take their medicine?" At first I thought that this person felt that without their medication there would be problems. I wondered, would pills help this person to feel safe? There was so much to interpret when I was already stressed about my sons' conditions.

Other times, the input of some family members can be harsh. "He needs his butt beat." "You should keep him at home." "What did the doctor say?" One time a family member actually said to my sons, "If you were my sons I would have put y'all in a home." After that insensitive comment, my youngest son shared with me his deep fear that I would do such a thing.

Siblings

Siblings can be protective or feel sympathy. Other times they may ridicule, bully or disassociate. They may feel sympathy for the parent. They may feel neglected and become overwhelmed with the burden of helping their sibling while forfeiting their own "normal" childhood. I'm sure that a sibling may even feel at fault for what the family as a whole is going through. No doubt they will feel anger, even at times hatred for the neurodivergent child, the parent, and even the disease itself.

AT HOME

As a mother with two children with ASD, I'm writing to express and expose some of the experiences that we as African Americans live through as families as we attempt to care for and seek help for our loved one. We endure so many concerns, limitations and fears. Here are only a few:

◆ What if I'm not parenting right?

◆ Am I not spanking enough?

◆ Is my form of discipline wrong?

◆ We already have enough working against us based on our color alone.

◆ This disease is going to isolate my child even more.

◆ Where does this come from?

◆ Does it change?

◆ What about their future?

◆ How do I help them become or at least look normal?

Knowing these societal and racial limitations, Black families try to mask, hide, minimize or even shut their eyes to their concerns for their ASD child:

◆ He is going to be like everybody else.

- ♦ We will compensate for their differences and unusualness.

- ♦ We will explain away his behavior with statements like, "He's shy, he doesn't talk much but he's really smart." "He's a little slow but he'll be fine." "He'll grow out of it."

- ♦ We will even avoid public places and large family gatherings to steer clear of reactions related to the child's behavior: rejection, embarrassment, questions, and well-meaning suggestions to name a few.

Tension increases at home with more distressing attacks: "You're coddling him." "Make him do this, do that." "You're just not a disciplinarian." My son was shamed for his gastrointestinal issues even at home (his father forced him to wash out his underwear in the toilet bowl).

My spouse and I, at the time, didn't have a clue how to manage this situation. We were guilty of going too far and allowing our anger and frustration to be expressed toward our son. I saw how the autism was pulling our marriage apart because of our ignorance, and finally, trying to stop my spouse from his abuse.

My son rode with me to work, which was his school as well. One morning after a very harsh experience with his dad forcing a pill down his throat, he asked me. "Does Jesus give hugs?" My heart sank, knowing how deeply sad he felt asking this question. He must have felt so alone and abandoned. I know I would. I felt helpless and guilty for not preventing such an event that hurt him like that.

I knew my son was having trouble with focus and staying on task, but outside of medication and discipline I had no idea what to do. Most of the answers and advice in the African American community was discipline (spanking). That wasn't helping. Then my own internal rage with my spouse and my sons' inability to conform led to me abusing my son.

I began to get help with counseling through Family Solutions, an agency that provides support for families. As for my spouse, I went as far as to contact children's services to get help about the abuse. I'm so remorseful about the ignorance and the inability to really help my son.

BEHAVIOR

ASD children display peculiar behavior in order to quell their anxiety in a neurotypical environment. Imagine being in a foreign country where you have no idea of how to speak the language, the culture and customs are totally unfamiliar to you, but you are expected to communicate with others, express your needs in an understandable way, and also have a productive day. People are speaking to you but you are not sure how to respond, and you don't always get the meaning of what they are saying. Maybe you all have a good laugh about it, but for an ASD child, simple sympathetic laughter can be interpreted as people laughing *at* him because he is out of his neurodivergent element.

Here is an example that may resonate. I used to have these dreams where I was somewhere in a public place, and I discovered that I had no clothes on. Boy was I so glad to wake up and discover that it was just a dream. The "wake up" for these children is going home at the end of the school day. My sons' entire day consisted of expectations to be or act neurotypically, but they did not know how. This is no different than your foreign country experience. The difference is you have the ability and ease to control your behavior that is accepted as normal. The ASD child does not have that gift that we take for granted.

ASD children use behaviors to cope with their own disorientation of their environment and their internal confusion which may include rocking, flapping their hands, hitting themselves, applying pressure on parts of their body, talking to themselves, repeating what others say.

My oldest son's preschool teacher complained that he would not diversify in play. He just played with cars and trucks and would misbehave when he was forced to leave that area for different play area.

His first grade teacher refused to allow my son to go on a field trip because he was having accidents that I learned later were caused by gastrointestinal problems. God bless Etolia, the parent that volunteered to escort him on the field trip to assist him if he had an accident.

My youngest son would often hit himself (punishing his head) calling himself, "stupid boy" for simply wearing clothes that other students weren't wearing. The same with my oldest son, who would cut his arm repeatedly, all of this due to frustration around communication issues and assumptions. ASD children are viewed by our society as distracting, embarrassing, or even suspecting evidence of abuse at home. I was once asked by a teacher if my seven-year-old son was involved in sexual behavior because he would keep one hand in his pocket. He was putting pressure on his leg. Of course I was outraged by such an assumption. I later learned that he was applying deep pressure helping him to manage his school environment. His book bag became increasingly heavy over time with his school materials and books that he liked to read. I didn't attempt to change his book bag because the contents were harmless. It was as though he needed the weight of his book bag to keep him from floating off the ground.

At Disney World, at the top of an air lift ride, was when I learned that my youngest son had a fear of heights. He was screaming, rocking the ride and trying to jump off. Terrified, he nor I had any idea that this fear even existed. Here again another incident of slow processing and communication issues for a person with autism.

So many questions I had, as any mother would, before

my son's diagnosis. Is my son bad? Is he not able to learn? What is wrong with him? Day after day I came to the same end with no answers. Both he and I were frustrated. No good reports from pre-school, kindergarten, first grade.

MAKING SOCIAL CONTACT

There are certain social awkward events I will never forget. My son went up to a gentleman after church and told him that he slept all the way through service. Another time when he was a teenager, he asked a mother, "You just had a baby, why are you still fat?"

This son has always been more forward socially (oddly so to be on the autism spectrum). He would frequently approach people with questions and statements. I learned to approach these people afterward with, "Well how did it go?" not knowing whether the conversation was pleasant or disturbing. I was never sure if he was going to compliment, question or criticize.

Another time when this same son was much older, he approached a church member who had not too long ago lost her husband. He tenderly put his hands on her shoulders, looked at her sincerely, then asked her, "How are you doing?" She told me about this experience and said it was like he knew how she was really feeling. She was deeply touched by his response to her.

CHILDCARE

It can be very difficult for the family/parent to get respite from the constant needs of the autistic child or children. Good childcare can help, but nothing will be perfect.

Even If you do secure childcare, interruptions will almost always occur because of increasing behavior problems. The child may become upset or act out because things are not the same as they are in their own home. Their complaint may be due to something as simple as a change in the weather or other circumstances that are out of the caregiver's control.

It may help to have the childcare provider to come to your home, or for the provider to take the child on an outing for a very short trip. A well-trained caregiver should understand that all conditions must be favorable as possible to the child, meaning a very low anxiety environment. Low anxiety situations can be a trial and error activity search that may involve a small group or individual, limiting the number of colors in their environment, low to no noise areas, neutral or natural smells, no fluorescent light but low lighting.

My personal experience with childcare providers has

involved situations where the provider has left early, needed to call the police because of threats of violence, violence toward the provider, or violence between my sons. Some agencies offered respite care, but unfortunately the funding for respite care would only be for "typical" babysitting but not providing trained persons that could work with autistic children.

Almost all providers didn't understand how to work with my sons. At any given moment, a "melt down" could send a provider into a state of terror with helpless attempts to calm the child down. Many care providers were personally offended by the social failure of these children.

My home was on speed dial with the police department because my sons would ultimately fight when a childcare provider was present. This was intimidating and scary as it was for me many times.

SCHOOL

Times are different now for schools with early intervention and more awareness of autism. During our time (my sons and myself) we heard, "he's not acting right. He won't participate. He only wants to do one thing. He keeps having accidents."

Autism is at epidemic proportions and schools are not that prepared to handle it. ASD is very difficult to handle from the perspective that it doesn't exist by itself. It comes with at least one comorbidity,[3] some of which are:

- attention deficit disorder
- attention deficit with hyperactivity disorder
- bipolar disorder
- heightened levels of anxiety
- sensory issues
- depression
- gastrointestinal issues
- obsessive compulsive disorder.
- Echolalia

---

[3] Children's Hospital of Philadelphia. https://www.chop.edu/news/autism-s-clinical-companions-frequent-comorbidities-asd

In my experience, my sons were high functioning and were placed with much lower functioning students, leading the educator to spend more time focusing on the lower functioning students. My sons fell behind academically, leaving high school without the preparedness for higher education.

I have met parents of ASD children my sons' age who have college degrees, and of course they are not African American. We were living in the same county within 15 miles of each other with a chasm of difference in achievement and opportunity between us.

Schools did and are still violating Individual Education Plans (IEP's) for special needs students leaving them without the tools they need to succeed in the future. Parents with the cash are landing costly lawsuits with these school systems. Yet when I pursued and paid with the little money I had for legal help for my children's violated IEP, it turned out to be an expensive run around with no tangible results that benefited my children at all.

"There is always a logical explanation." "Logical explanation" is the code language for the chasm that existed between the Caucasian American disabled child and the African American disabled child which is habitually ignored and devalued. I was completely ignorant of strategies and options. I was addressed with statements like, maybe I should have tried "this" or "that" to achieve different outcomes for my sons. I didn't even know the "this" or "that" even existed.

Charter schools are on the rise specializing with students on the autism spectrum. There is more state funding for an autistic child than any other disabled child. However, the very stringent training for working with these students is rarely met, because state regulations for "highly qualified educators" in charter schools is more relaxed. Keep in mind that charter schools are more likely to be, "for profit" schools as a business model.

The frequent occurrence of autism[4] would prompt me to think that there would be just cause to have one out of three schools in each school district set up to work with these students' needs. These students' various superior abilities

---

[4] https://www.cdc.gov/autism/data-research/index.html 1 per 68 in 2010, now 1 per 36 in 2020.

would be a great benefit to that district's local community. They tend to have one or more abilities that supersede that of students of the same age and experience. Autism has given us some of our most valued inventions, theories, philosophies and much more.[5]

---

[5] "Code breakers" was a term coined by Hans Asperger. He used this label for his atypical, institutionalized patients in an attempt to prevent their annihilation by Nazi Germany. It was then he began to observe and realize their superior academic abilities.

SCHOOL SOCIAL LOSSES

ASD children experience many losses at school. They often miss out on awards like "citizen of the month," and invitations to classmates birthday parties.

One of my most painful experiences was when the boys were very young. We went from hosting birthday parties with a half a dozen or more children in attendance, then to never being invited to any of their birthday parties. I believe I wouldn't have felt worse if my heart was literally ripped out of my chest. No child deserves that kind of disappointment. I would have pondered suicide just as much as they did if I wasn't so needed by them.

When my youngest son was in the second grade at a private school, he invited his entire class to his birthday party. A half hour past the time the party should have begun, he asked where everybody was. I asked him if he gave everyone an invite. He responded with "yes." No one came. To ease the situation, I called a neighbor whose son did not go to the same school as mine, and he came for a quiet evening of play with him.

My oldest son experienced the same as an adult. He

invited many friends with whom he associated within his community to my home, where I would host the party preparing food for his guests. No one came. He was devastated. Later that evening he overdosed on his medication and was then hospitalized.

Peer Bullying

Bullying occurs from just about every direction: from students, teachers and even perceived bullying. Much of the bullying from peers goes unreported by the ASD child. The child's lack of social understanding of what is appropriate or inappropriate makes it difficult to identify an offense. Some examples: "You're weird." My son was goaded by students into saying things to others that were inappropriate just for laughs. Other students even pressured him into giving them his personal belongings by saying that he owed them. They physically hurt him as if it was a game. The autistic student doesn't process that bullies are not friends. They don't possess social cues, nor do they communicate well about how they feel. So they are left with not knowing whether this is how life really is supposed to be with their peers.

At a private school, my son accidentally damaged something belonging to another student. It was replaced immediately. However the student insisted that he pay her money repeatedly. He kept returning home needing more money for lunch that was already paid. He finally told me about the student demanding his lunch money causing him to feel remorseful to pay some kind of penance.

At another private school my son was told by some neurotypical students to say some very inappropriate things to an adult. Because of his social inabilities he was unaware of the inappropriateness of the statement, thus not understanding that these boys weren't trying to be his friend, it was about getting a laugh. And of course the crime fit his gender and color. Those boys didn't look like him. Neither did the girl at the other private school.

Even as adults, my sons have trouble identifying appropriate and inappropriate behavior with their peers, many times still being bullied. ASD children are very literal and they take what you say as what you mean without exceptions. For example, I taught my son not to physically fight others. He followed that directive even when a group of his peers tried to steal his bike from him. They hit him repeatedly. A police officer saw and stopped the offense. He returned home and proudly announced that he didn't fight back as the boys kept hitting him to get him to give them his bike.

Teacher Bullying

Teachers can target stimming behavior (rocking/pressing down on oneself/repetitive movement) as misbehavior. They can refuse to follow IEP directives, not allowing extended time for assignments due to processing speed of the student), not abbreviating assignments (because of focus and anxiety issues). I was told that abbreviated tests were unfair to other students.

This misunderstood disability has lent itself to me using visual scenarios with sarcasm to express my anger for the ignorance of others. "So, I guess it is unfair to the walking public to have ramps for the wheelchair bound public?"

I experienced constant battles with teachers not willing to follow the IEP for my sons. In the teachers' defense (I am a teacher as well), there was little to no training for teachers in order to address educational instruction for autism spectrum students. I often became very angry with the teachers (my colleagues in the same school system) who refused to follow my sons' IEP, which schools are legally bound to follow. I said many times, "If you refuse to do this for me as your colleague, what are you doing with the parent that does not understand this document and may be struggling with the same disability?"

Academic Bullying

ASD students often have superior intelligence in one of two academic areas, reading or math. This sometimes results in the assumption that both academic areas are strong, or that both academic areas are weak. Thus instructional focus on these content areas may not be well developed. It is often assumed that students of superior intelligence in either of these content areas are perceived as competent in social situations. Ultimately these students wind up being grouped with lower functioning students, so their needs for success aren't addressed well.

My sons weren't well-prepared to transition past high school graduation. My sons functioned high enough to be college students, however, a full load in college would be second to impossible for them to handle. No financial support was available for part time ASD college students, nor was there academic support to fit their specific learning needs. The lower functioning students were targeted or picked up by transition agencies/groups for technical training or employment due to their lower scores on graduation test.

COMMUNITY AGENCIES

There are some great community agencies that assist families of children with disabilities. Unfortunately finding the resources can be very difficult if you don't know the right people or the right questions to ask. In the African American community many of these resources are hidden from us, or we just didn't know the "right questions" to ask. There are many success stories that involve Caucasian families that African Americans have not experienced due to a system that we all (White and Black) are trapped in. This system has historically red lined our Black community in housing, jobs, schools, etc. Regardless of our many skin tones, it is clear that as African Americans we must be more skillful, more intelligent, more educated to achieve the economic position that equals or rivals that of our white counterpart. This is more than abundantly true for African American families of autistic children seeking resources for our loved ones.

Tamika, a mother I know well, sought help for her son via calls and letters to an agency that helps the disabled community. She was refused services for her son repeatedly. Upon reading her letters, I surmised that the language she used in her letters did not move the agency to address her son's needs. Consequently, she had a hard time understanding what they were conveying back to her. They were repeatedly blowing off all her requests. This state agency left her family with no help to care for their son who needed constant supervision. This caused her and her husband to work separate work shifts in order to keep their son safe. This ultimately affected their marriage relationship negatively. Their son could easily figure out a complex lock system to get out of the house, and this young man was a "runner." Once out of the reach of his parents, he would run without caution, subjecting himself to danger on their busy street and unknown places, causing his parents to chase him until they physically caught him. He never responded to their calls to him.

    This is one among many stories of a lack of supportive resources that are often "restricted" and "out of reach" for African American families. I can fairly state that the fight for services for our African American children with autism are not only hidden, it takes repeated and constant documentation to get a response for help.

In my own home, one son constantly moved and the other son was over stimulated by his movement. This resulted in the use of force by one son to stifle the other. As time went on, the son with constant movement began collecting items to use as a weapon to protect himself if he was attacked by his brother. My sons had to be constantly watched to protect them from hurting each other. This typically meant that I had virtually no private time when we were all together. So preparing meals and using the restroom became very challenging. I needed to have at least one present with me when we were home together. Using the phone, watching television and reading was pretty much nonexistent most of the time for me. In addition to constant surveillance of the two, there was a sensory diet that needed to be followed several times a day with my youngest son.

With all the facts concerning violence, sensory diet and constant surveillance, my application for a disability waiver was refused. This waiver would have provided an opportunity for in home support. The agency insisted that I could administer the sensory diet while fixing meals, helping with homework, keeping the sons from hurting each and preparing for the next day of work, and school. All at once.

As I continued to request in-home support services repeatedly, I was told again and again that no funds were available. Finally, I requested a board review and brought in a White female advocate named Patty (who worked for the same state funded agency in a different county) to join me in this board review. She supported my claims of repeated violence in my home due to the differences in each son. Finally, with Patty's help, we convinced the board to help my family.

Specialized childcare for respite was simply unavailable. These parents don't just need babysitters. Even in teen years these youngsters need specialized care. They need someone that can anticipate a meltdown before it happens, diffuse it, then redirect the one who isn't having a meltdown, while still completing any task at hand.

I leaned on family members like any parent would. I also hired sitters when I could not be with my sons due to work demands. During those times I almost always received calls of a crisis with my sons.

The police became very familiar with our address as it

related to violence between my sons or other crisis incidents involving runaway reports.

My neighbor that I affectionately refer to as "sis" did not speak to me for a long time after moving across from me. Finally one day she approached me to ask when the city was going to collect the leaves that were to be put on the median strip. Much later as we became close, I asked her why it took so long for her to warm up to me. She said she didn't understand what was going on with my sons. The guys were in their teens at the time, and both would fight or threaten each other. She told me how afraid she was when she saw the youngest chasing the oldest down the street with a knife, and seeing the police at my house a few times.

NOW: THE HEART OF THE MATTER
A Mother's Heart/Hurt.

I didn't know! I didn't understand! Why he wouldn't hug family members. Why he walked on his toes. Why his child care providers would complain about his focus only on one area of play. Why he would just fall out when he didn't "seemly" get his way. My need was immense to find a childcare provider that would be sensitive and responsive to an autistic child.

Finally I found a psychological test to learn that our son had some superior intelligence but some really low areas. No diagnosis yet because no one in our local area was knowledgeable of this new diagnosis. First he was given medication for ADHD (attention deficit hyperactivity disorder). Oh how my heart hurts just thinking back on the mismanagement of this process. We (doctors and myself) just didn't know!! Then the school took the abusive notion that he was viewed as just being rebellious and defiant.

Then came my second son. The abuse toward our older son started to internalize, and he started lashing out on his baby brother. Needless to say it wasn't long before the marriage fell apart along with other issues Our youngest son became hyper-vigilant as a result of the abuse and the violence coming from his brother, and so the cycle of abuse continued stretching back to both of our childhood experiences.

By the time my oldest son was in third grade and my youngest son was in kindergarten, the need for a diagnosis finally came to my attention. A college student who was doing a student classroom experience in my class began to share with me about her brother. She was the first to mention Asperger Syndrome to me. Her stories about her brother helped me to further investigate what could be going on with my oldest son. She told me that one of her adult brother's awkwardness was how he interacted with strangers in public as if he had known them for a very long time, carrying on long conversations with them, yet at the same time being unaware that he had been urinating on himself at the same time. This young woman's willingness to share such private information changed the trajectory of my children's lives.

Interestingly, my adult son, too, engages in long personal conversations with complete strangers to this day. He may ask if they are married to the person they are with and even predict that they will be married at a designated time. Depending on their response he would say, "So you two are just friends with benefits."

Hunting for services was at first a crap shoot. First neurology to address ADD and ADHD. Medication that was right for my son was difficult to discover and in retrospect, I don't know what damage may have occurred or is still to be discovered. One medicine had my son hallucinating that bugs were all over him. I later found out that medicine "vacation or breaks" on the weekend were the chemical equivalent of shaking a baby causing brain damage. Because of our geographic location, we had to travel a minimum of an hour to find real medical, psychological, neurological, psychiatric and homeopathic help.

My sons' needs became more and more critical as one contemplated suicide as early as eight years old. One evening when he was supposed to walk home from a neighbor's house after I got home from work, but it was taking far too long for him to get home. Finally when I headed out to comb the neighborhood looking for him, there he was at the front door telling me that he was taking so long because he was going to jump in front of a car to kill himself. These suicidal ideologies continue on to this day.

The search for resources continued to challenge us. We travelled for medical treatment on an average of two to three times weekly. We were leaving early for school and medical appointments, then returning home well after dark to eat and head to bed, then repeat that pattern the next day.

I realized that I had to make a major change when my youngest son whined, "Do we have another appointment today?" The anguish in his voice made it clear to me that something had to change. So the following school year I decided to job share, which was basically part time. This caused a major economic impact on my income with many financial limitations. There was no eating out. Regular meals were tuna noodle casserole, spaghetti, chicken pot pie, BBQ beef round-up and meat loaf.

How a mother feels

I know that my sons needed friends, but the school and church setting wasn't the draw for them. I learned quickly that the neighborhood could and would respond to my sons as they played with fun toys that attracted other boys in the area. I purchased gaming systems and other items that other boys in the neighborhood would be drawn to come and play with my guys. I planned a birthday celebration for my oldest son that involved dinner and a movie with two friends of his choice since parties weren't successful.

Finally when he was 18, a church member approached me and asked me to make sure he could come to her daughter's birthday party. I was overwhelmed with the thought that someone truly wanted his company at their party after all these years of not one invitation from anyone. I just cried.

My sons have really shaped me into the person I am now. Many stories of them with their literal understanding, and perseverating on various topics, have been some of the most enlightening experiences and sometime just down right hilarious.

Once my son and I were at the doctor's office and the doctor wanted to speak to me alone and asked him to wait in the waiting room. Knowing that he loved to read, the doctor asked him what he would do in the waiting room that was filled with books and magazines. My son replied, "Wait."

I was late putting on my seat belt one day with my youngest son in the car, and because it was taking me too long, he finally said, "Just die then."

Another time he and I were riding in the car, he was going on and on about some topic that I wasn't interested in, and my thoughts were occupied with something else. I told him that I wasn't able to listen to him at that time. He responded with, "I don't care" and continued on ad nauseam.

This same son perseverated about different things. He complained that he needed to see a doctor about his penis because it wasn't growing. We went to see his pediatrician, and she told him that he was growing just fine and there were no issues with his growth. A little while later he insisted on seeing another doctor. He said, "That was a female doctor, I want to see a man, I want to see a urologist." That doctor confirmed that he was growing just fine and there were no concerns about his development. Of course he was not finish perseverating[6] because shortly after that appointment, I arrived home to be greeted at the door by my oldest son saying, "Mom, Male Enhancement keeps calling here and I think he's been calling them."

My oldest son was very good at sticking to the rules. He came home from the corner store and said that he found a twenty dollar bill on the sidewalk. I asked, "Where is it honey?" He said, "I put it back where I found it." This was the same as how he responded to the boys trying to steal his bike. He didn't hit back based on my rule "No fighting." I failed to include, "unless a few boys are hitting you to take your bike." Dah! I should have told him.

I sometimes wish I knew or could experience what it is like to have a more neurotypical child. I envied others because their children started where mine did but their outcomes are so vastly different. I know this is true for any parent. I just believe that there is a "moccasin" experience, to "walk in another's shoes" that can only be related to in that way.

---

[6] Perseveration is a common symptom of autism spectrum disorder (ASD) characterized by the persistent repetition of thoughts, behaviors, or actions.

DIVINE GUIDANCE

A mother's path to healing comes from the Most High's hand on my sons' lives. From the beginning, he gave me Rilinda, the college student who worked in my classroom for her student experience course. Her openness to share such personal experiences about her ASD brother was priceless. She led me to exploring my son's issues.

The Sunday school teachers, Brian and Allen, as well as mentors Gerald, Edgar and my brother, took a great interest in my sons despite their disabilities. I created a "Black Bar Mitzvah" for my oldest son. I asked five men to come over for a brief visit after Sunday service to speak into his life when he was turning 13 years of age. To my surprise these men were deeply honored to do such a thing. They came well prepared with written notes in hand to speak to my son. I was overwhelmed by their love and support for him.

Afterward, three of the men stood outside near their cars for over an hour. They talked extensively about a mentoring program for young boys that they were trying to get started. The men were inspired that their time with my son was a clear sign that they needed to get this program officially off the ground and for my son to be included in the pilot program.

The "Rites of Passage" program was created. It has been a true gift to both of my sons. This positive "male life experience" that I could not provide holds a lifetime value. My sons over time have often attached themselves to positive male groups for advice and camaraderie that wasn't easily attainable due to their social awkwardness.

I'm indebted to a home health agency owned by Souleatha that deliberately sought out male providers to work with my sons. Her wisdom about the needs of my sons is exemplary.

My involvement with Aspie (a group of parents with autistic children) led to me working directly with another mother, Sharlene, in this journey which led to a deeper understanding of the disease. Together we produced a program to assist teachers and parents on how to work with autistic children like ours.

This relationship led to a string of connections. An attorney who himself had autism pointed me to the Jane Polly show where the North Star Service Dog Agency was featured.

From there came our beloved service dog "Blue." After getting this beautiful standard poodle, my youngest son finally began to have eye contact when folks addressed him about his dog Blue. Later he and Blue became stars in an episode of "Good Dog," a Lucky Duck production with Linda Ellerbee on the TV program about types of service dogs.

We have been favored to say the least in this blindfolded journey through many troublesome events with equal amounts of uplifting navigations to an ever changing path.

My sons are now adults and living independently with support from their service support administrator from Summit Developmentally Delayed Agency.

At this point, and from my perspective, survival is their highest level of success as Black men in these United States of America versus the counter culture who may have vastly different success that can be simply unavailable to children that look like mine.

Friends and family would often ask me; "How are the guys?" I went from saying "They're ok" to, "They've got a good mom" to, "I'm sure heaven is my home because I'm living in hell now," to silence; I stopped talking to friends or family so the subject didn't have a chance to come up.

The pain of this disease has left many scars that have made me the human that I am. I am very conflicted between the absence having neurotypical children in my life, and the pleasure of being chosen to raise such incredible human beings. They are gifted with superior intelligence in the area of language, and they have great compassion for others. They are all this, but I will never forget the terrible pain and scars they have suffered for being socially misunderstood, misread and constantly bullied just because they are different.

Of course the future is unknown for all of us. What I do know and believe is that autism is categorized as "developmentally delayed." I believe that my sons are still developing. They are now in their late 20's and mid 30's. I did all that I knew to do to teach them, support them, fight for them and show up in every way that I could. I love these guys with all my heart, sweat and tears.

What I have instilled in them shows up repeatedly and is seen as well by others: *"Every time I see your son he is so respectful and always acknowledges me."* I'm NOT OK with autism for what it has done to our lives, but I have to let it be OK for our future. Our scars that come from numerous hurtful wounds show proof of my Healer and my God in whom I'm committed to trusting in for my sons' future.

Things to Consider

- Constantly let your love know that they are beautiful and blessed.
- Get past STIGMAS!
- Stand in the Gap for your love one.
- Start EARLY! Start EARLY!
- Parents take YOURSELF out of IT
- It's about "What can you do for the success of your child."
- Keep going; get more and more information that supports your child.
- Others give up but YOU DON'T!
- Push OPEN closed doors
- There is help everywhere; Don't STOP
- Get your church family involved in your child's needs.

Made in the USA
Coppell, TX
16 January 2026

68222620R00031